Homemade Herbal Tea Recipes Using Nature to Heal, Maintain Health, and Safely Lose Weight

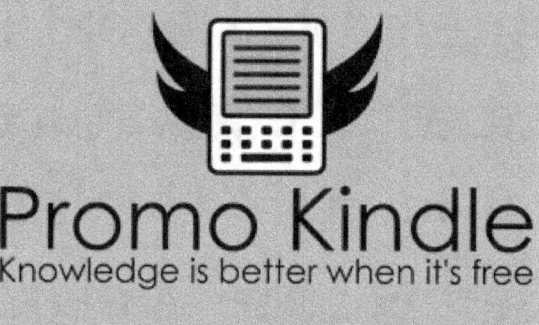

Table of Contents

Health ailments & remedies

Peppermint Tea

Ingredients:
- 1 handful mint leaves
- Hot water

Directions: Start by chopping up the leaves, add the tea to your tea kettle, add hot water, you can add honey or sugar or any other sweetener. This will help with stomach aches and headaches.

Ginger Root tea

Ingredients:
- 1 chunk ginger root
- Hot water

Directions: add fresh ginger root and peel grate and at to tea kettle. Pour water and let sit or boil for 5-8 minutes.

Honey Throat Tea

Ingredients:
- 2 T coconut oil
- 2 T raw honey
- 1 tsp. ground cinnamon

Direction: Mix everything but your water until you have a paste like substance. This is more like a paste than a tea, but it can be boiled with water, strained and turned into great tea as well.

Lemons make lemonade

Ingredients:
- Lemon juice
- 3 T raw honey
- Water
- Lemon slices

Directions: whisk honey and lemon together and dilute as needed with water, can be served warm or cold.

Flu- Away tea

Ingredients:
- 2 C chicken stock
- 1 tsp ground turmeric
- 1/8 tsp cinnamon
- Black peppercorns
- 2 cardamom
- 1 fresh ginger
- 2 tsp minced garlic

Directions: Add everything but the last ingredients to a boil then simmer for around 6 minutes or so. Strain and add garlic once the cooled enough, and drink up!

Basic Cold & Flu tea

Ingredients:
- 4 slices ginger with skin
- ½ T minced garlic
- Cayenne powder
- Green tea
- Honey of taste
- Milk

Directions: Bring ginger and garlic to a boil then let simmer for just under 30 minutes. Use ginger to steep the tea, add cayenne pepper, this is to help induce sweating to break fevers, add honey to taste, or preference, add milk and if you can drink 3-4 cups per bed.

Garlic fever reducer

Ingredients:
- 3 cloves garlic
- 3 slices ginger
- Mason jar
- Lemon
- Water

Directions: In Mason jar add 3 cloves garlic and 3 sliced of ginger, cover and let steep for 20-25 minutes add 1 ½ lemons and honey to taste. Strain herbs and serve. Try and drink this warm.

Herbal Tea for Weight Loss recipes

Lavender iced tea

Ingredients:
- 1 ½ tsp dried lavender
- 4 tea bags

Directions: heat up 1 ½ C water in kettle or sauce pan and let simmer, remove from heat and add tea bags and lavender let sit for 5 minutes, strain and let cool. You can add ice to an Ice pitcher or store in refrigerator.

Green Tea smoothie

Ingredients:
- 2 ½ C frozen mango
- ¾ C yogurt
- ¼ C honey
- Peeled and sliced kiwi
- ½ C baby spinach chopped
- 2 T Bottled great tea
- 2 T water
- 2 C ice

Directions: In blender add everything together and blend until smoothie texture and pour into 1-2-4 glasses. This is a weight loss green tea smoothie

Cranberry green tea spritzer

Ingredients:
- 4 tea bags
- ½ C cranberry juice
- 3 C seltzer
- 1/3 C sugar
- 1/3 C water

Directions: boil water and sugar until sugar dissolves completely, add tea bags and let sit for 2 minutes. Remove bags, add cranberry juice. Add seltzer last and serve.

Blue Green tea smoothie

Ingredients:
- 2 green tea bags
- 2 C fresh blueberries
- 12 oz. non-fat yogurt (vanilla)
- 2 T crushed almonds
- 2 T flaxseed
- ¾ C water
- Ice

Directions: Start by boiling water and adding tea bags and let sit for about 4 minutes. Remove tea bags and let water/tea chill overnight or for at least 6-8 hours. Add everything else to blueberries and blend, pour once reaches smoothie texture.

Ingredients:
- 8 green tea bags
- 4 C boiling water
- ½ C sweetener

Directions: Take boiling water and add tea bags and let steep for 5 minutes. Carefully remove tea bags, and add sweetener and wait for that to dissolve. Ready when room temperature. Could be served as iced tea or hot tea.

Herbal Tea recipes for sleep

Digestive Tea

Ingredients:
- 1 part spearmint leaves
- 1/8 part dried licorice root

Directions: Mix the two roots together store in a glass Mason jar or similar jar. Use 1 T per 1 C hot water

Adrenal tea

Ingredients:
- 1 C ashwagandha root
- 1 C shatavari root
- 1 C tulsi holy basil
- ½ Cinnamon chips

Directions: Mix everything together in one bowl, this will serve for more than just one glass of hot tea. Use 2 T per medium saucepan or tea kettle. Boil 1-2 C of water OVER the herbs and allow it to simmer for 15-20 minutes.

Winter Chai

Ingredients:
- 4 C Darjeeling tea
- 1 C cinnamon chips
- ¼ C ground nutmeg
- 1 C ginger
- ½ C cloves
- 4 vanilla beans, cut up

Directions: Mix the ingredients together in a large bowl, you will scoop up tea as you use it. Boil 1 C of water to 1 tsp of tea mix

Tea for Women

Uterine tonic tea

Ingredients:

- Alfalfa
- Red clover leaf
- Raspberry leaf
- Nettle
- Yarrow
- Oat straw
- Fennel seed
- Rose petals
- Lemon balm
- Orange peel
- Hibiscus flowers
- Peppermint
- Vitex

Directions: 1 tsp of each herb and one C hot boiling water. And serve

Ingredients:
- Chamomile
- Skullcap
- Lemon balm
- Lavender

Directions: Mix 1 tsp each herb plus 1 C hot water.

Ingredients:
- Red raspberry infusion
- Nettle tea
- Chamomile infusion

Directions: start with 1 oz. to 1 C boiling water

Baby Teething tea

Ingredients:
- 1 tsp. chamomile
- 1 tsp. lavender
- 1 tsp. catnip
- 1 tsp. skullcap
- 1 tsp oat straw
- 1 tsp rose hips
- 1 tsp. red clover
- 1 tsp. cloves

Directions: add ½ oz. of each herb and store in a jar, as before, and make 1-2 tsp. of added mixture per 1 C of water.

After school snack tea

Ingredients:
- Chamomile
- St. John's Wort
- Pinch of lavender

Directions: Add about 1 tsp of the first two ingredients and 1/8 tsp of lavender and boil 1 C water per tsp of mixed herbs. Boil. You can add honey to taste if you would like or fresh lemon.

Herbal Chai

Ingredients:
- 16 cloves
- 16 cardamom pods
- 2 sticks cinnamon
- Ginger root
- 2 tsp. fennel seeds
- 2 T rooibos
- 5 C water
- 2 C milk
- Honey

Directions: You need to smash the herbs, you want a paste like substance, add herbs to water and let simmer around 15-20 minutes. Add milk and take off the heat and add rooibos. Steep for 8-10 minutes.

Energy Tea shake

Ingredients:
- 2 tea bag green tea
- 2 T dried maca root
- 1 C hemp seed milk
- 1 tsp raw honey
- 1 tsp bee pollen

Directions: brew up your favorite tea (the green tea mentioned in the ingredients) in blender add all remaining ingredients, and pour and serve.

Ginseng energy tea

Ingredients:
- 2 T fresh ginger root tea, grated
- 24 oz. spring water
- 2 lemons, freshly squeezed
- 20 drops ginseng root extract
- 2 T coconut sugar
- 1 tsp blackstrap molasses

Directions: Add grated ginseng in water and simmer for about 30 minutes, and you will know because your kitchen will smell awesome. Strain into jar add rest of ingredients, and stir well, and serve. This can be hot or cold.

Green tea with lemon

Ingredients:
- 1-2 Green tea bag
- Struvia
- ½ lemon

Directions: This is really simple, but you can add the tea bags to 4 C boiling water and let set for about 30-45 minutes, let water simmer so it doesn't evaporate. Add Struvia drops in your tea cup add lemon and pour tea into glass.

Honey Lavender Tea

Ingredients:
- 1-2 tea bags (your preference)
- 1 T honey
- 1 tsp lavender
- 4 C water

Directions: Boil your water with the tea bags, and let simmer, add remaining ingredients and serve hot